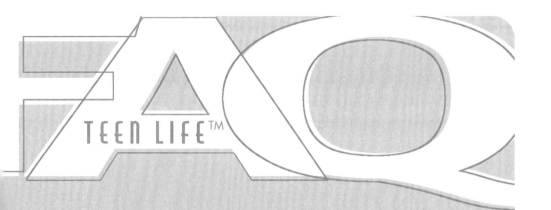

FREQUENTLY ASKED QUESTIONS ABOUT

Migraines and Headaches

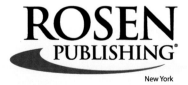

Allan B.
Cobb

ROSEN
PUBLISHING®
New York

Published in 2009 by The Rosen Publishing Group, Inc.
29 East 21st Street, New York, NY 10010
www.rosenpublishing.com

Copyright © 2009 by The Rosen Publishing Group, Inc.

First Edition

Library of Congress Cataloging-in-Publication Data

Cobb, Allan B.
Frequently asked questions about migraines and headaches/
Allan B. Cobb. — 1st ed.
      p. cm. — (FAQ: Teen life)
Includes bibliographical references and index.
ISBN-13: 978-1-4042-1814-7 (library binding)
1. Migraine—Juvenile literature. 2. Headache—Juvenile
literature. I. Title.
RC392.C62 2009
616.8'4912—dc22

                                                    2007049652

Manufactured in the United States of America

Contents

Chapter one

WHAT ARE MIGRAINE HEADACHES?

Headaches are common. Nearly everyone gets them at one time or another. However, not everyone gets the most severe type of headache, which is called a migraine.

Migraine is a condition of recurring severe headaches that are often accompanied by nausea and vomiting. People usually call them migraine headaches or simply migraines.

A migraine is not just a bad headache but a certain type of headache. True migraines do not happen every day. Some people get migraines only once or twice a year. Other people have migraines as often as ten times a month. In adults, migraine pain is usually on one side of the head, but in young people, it is often on both sides. During the migraine, the person may be sensitive to lights and noise. The person may also have a sensation just prior to

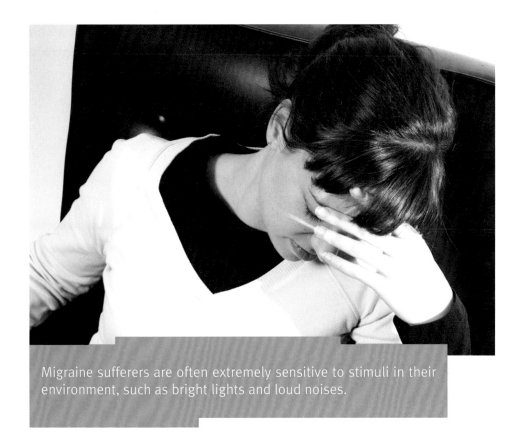

Migraine sufferers are often extremely sensitive to stimuli in their environment, such as bright lights and loud noises.

the onset of a migraine such as smelling burning rubber or seeing blinking lights. These symptoms are called auras.

You may have heard people use the term "migraine" for an extremely painful headache. Remember, though, that when you talk about having a migraine, you are talking about a specific type of headache, not just a severely aching head.

In short, headaches manifest themselves in many ways. The more information you can provide your doctor about the circumstances in which you experience the headache and the other symptoms occurring with it, the more easily your doctor can diagnose the type of headache you are experiencing. Then he or she can suggest appropriate treatment.

Who Gets Migraines?

Experts say that twenty-four million Americans (eighteen million women and six million men) get migraine headaches. Between 50 to 75 percent of young people get headaches now and then. Between 5 and 10 percent of these headaches are migraines. This number may be an underestimate because many people take over-the-counter pain relievers for migraines—or simply suffer.

Migraine headaches may start as early as age two or even younger. The frequency of migraines tends to peak during the teen years and early twenties. Another peak occurs in people between the ages of thirty-five and forty-five. The older people get, the less likely they are to have migraine attacks.

In their early years, boys and girls get migraine headaches in about equal numbers. But after puberty, young women pull ahead. Experts believe hormonal changes related to a woman's menstrual cycle may trigger migraine headaches. That is one explanation for women having three times as many migraine headaches as men.

One of the strange things about migraine headaches is that what happens before the headache may be almost as important as during the headache itself. Why? There are two main reasons. Knowing what comes before the headache helps doctors to classify and treat the headache. Also, various kinds of pain medication are more effective if a person takes these medications as soon as possible, before the headache takes hold.

The word "prodrome" describes the stage before a headache—the warning period. As much as a day or more before a headache, some young people describe feelings that may be warnings of an oncoming headache, such as irritability, tiredness, and depression.

The aura is another experience that occurs even closer to the onset of a migraine (thirty to sixty minutes prior). The word "aura" means a sensation of something more to come. Only about 20 percent of those with migraine headaches have auras, but an aura can be as dramatic as fireworks on the Fourth of July.

Auras are often highly visual. People see flashing lights, shimmering or zig-zagging lines, or blind spots. The "Alice-in-Wonderland" syndrome describes visual problems in which large figures turn into small ones and small ones into large ones. Some people experience numbness or tingling in various parts of their bodies during an aura. Others have trouble speaking. For some reason, the smell of burning rubber is a particularly common aura.

Different Types of Migraines

According to the International Headache Society, there are two major migraine classifications: migraine without aura—the most common type of migraine—and migraine with aura. In trying to classify your headache and make an accurate diagnosis, your doctor will probably ask you the following questions:

Over a period of time, have you had at least five of these attacks?

Have the headaches lasted from four hours to three days? (In young people, a migraine headache may be as short as an hour.)

The doctor's next questions will have to do with how the headache feels to you.

Is the headache on one side only? (The answer for adult migraine sufferers will likely be yes, but for young people, a migraine headache may be on both sides.)

Does the headache pound or pulsate?

Is the headache very painful? In other words, on a scale of 1 to 10, is it at least an 8, 9, or 10?

Does it hurt more with physical activity?

For a doctor to consider your headache a migraine, the answer would have to be yes to at least two of the above questions. A doctor's next set of questions will concern other physical feelings that go along with migraine headaches.

When you have a headache, do you feel sick to your stomach? Do you throw up?

During the headache, are you sensitive to lights or noise?

Those who have true migraines will answer yes to one or both of these questions. If you have migraines with aura, mention the sensations you experience to your doctor. An accurate classification of your type of migraine will make treatment more effective.

Some uncommon headaches are even more complicated than those already mentioned. These rare headaches not only hurt but can cause symptoms that can be very scary.

Basilar artery migraine: This type of headache is most likely to affect teenage women. The sufferer may vomit and experience visual problems, dizziness, vertigo, trouble walking, and even loss of consciousness. Unlike the usual migraine headache, this one may hurt in the back of the head. The basilar artery runs atop the brainstem and is near the cerebellum, which may account for the vertigo and balance difficulties.

Hemiplegic migraine: Scientists have found that this type of headache may be hereditary, or passed down from one generation to another. That is why it is sometimes called familial hemiplegic migraine. The hemiplegia (paralysis of one side of the body) or hemiparesis (weakness of one side of the body) at the onset of this headache sometimes lasts well after the headache ends.

Confusional migraine: A confused mental state, including possible amnesia, or memory loss, is the hallmark of the confusional migraine, which is more common in boys. The sufferer may become restless and disoriented. Afterward, he or she may have no memory of the headache.

Ophthalmoplegic migraine: The double vision and other eye problems that accompany this rare headache may last a long time after the headache is gone.

Cluster headache: Another rare variety of headache is the cluster headache. Some say it is a migraine and some say it isn't, but people describe it as extremely painful. However, it rarely appears in people under twenty.

What Causes Migraines?

Scientists believe that migraine headaches have strong genetic roots. At least 70 percent of those with migraine headaches have a close relative (usually a parent or grandparent) who also has migraines.

Nervous System

Although no one knows the exact reason why people get migraines, it appears that those who get migraines have a mild instability of the nervous system and blood vessels. During a migraine attack, a "spreading depression" of tiny electrical currents travels from the back to the front of the brain. This current can cause the blood vessels in the brain to tighten and deliver less blood. The migraine sufferer may experience an aura, blurry vision, or dizziness from this partial blood shutdown. When the blood vessels rebound, they dilate, or swell up. This may cause them to leak a small amount of pain-causing chemicals into the skin of the scalp.

The structures in the head that can hurt are the nerves, the blood vessels, and the covering of the brain, not the brain itself. A large nerve (the fifth, or trigeminal, nerve) on the underside of the brain senses chemical and blood vessel changes. At the same time, serotonin, a neurotransmitter that carries messages from nerve to nerve, is also involved in the

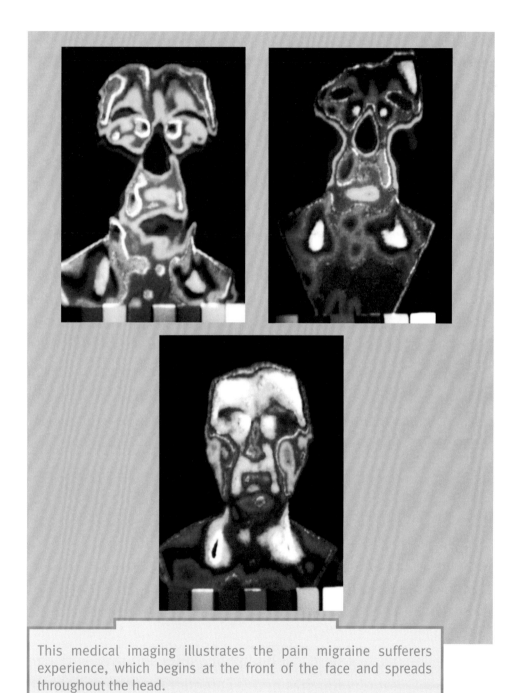

This medical imaging illustrates the pain migraine sufferers experience, which begins at the front of the face and spreads throughout the head.

transmission of pain. A lack of serotonin can make the blood vessels swell or become larger, causing the throbbing pain of a migraine.

Tension Headaches

People who have frequent headaches often have more than one type of headache. Sometimes one kind of headache merges into another.

Most headaches are not migraines. Probably the most common of all headaches is the tension headache. People used to call tension headaches "stress headaches" or "muscle-contraction" headaches. Although stress may play a role in the development of a tension headache, it is not the only cause.

Tension headaches often feel as if a belt or a piece of elastic has been pulled tightly around the scalp. Physical activity doesn't seem to make this pain any worse. The head doesn't throb as it would with a migraine, and the person doesn't usually vomit or feel nauseated. When a tension headache makes the person sensitive to bright lights and certain noises, it may be hard to distinguish from a migraine. In fact, some researchers believe that tension headaches are a less intense form of migraine. The headache can last from one hour to several days. Doctors classify tension headaches in two ways:

Episodic

Episodic means repeatedly, or happening over and over. A doctor may classify your headaches in this category if you experience a couple of headaches most weeks but fewer than fifteen

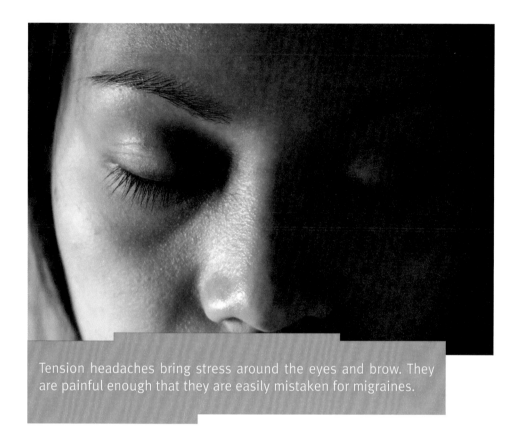

Tension headaches bring stress around the eyes and brow. They are painful enough that they are easily mistaken for migraines.

episodes a month. Most people with episodic tension headaches get relief from over-the-counter pain medications, ice packs to the head, naps, and/or relaxation exercises.

Chronic Tension Headaches/Chronic Daily Headaches

Imagine having a headache every day of your life. This kind of pain can really get to you. Those with chronic daily headaches have discomfort every day (or almost every day) for six months or longer. Over-the-counter pain relievers do not help. In fact, some pain medications can even make a headache worse, causing a "rebound" headache. A person with any kind of headache who takes too much pain medication can experience the rebound syndrome. When this happens, it is recommended that sufferers stop taking all pain medications.

Other Causes of Headaches

Other types of headaches are categorized according to their cause and whether or not the cause is life-threatening. Chances are you will never experience the causes of these types of headaches. They are serious but rare.

Brain Tumors

Brain tumors cause many of the same symptoms as migraines, but over time, a brain tumor headache will hurt more, will last longer, and is not likely to go away. If you have never had a serious headache and suddenly experience this kind of pain, you should see a doctor right away. A headache accompanied by seizures, vomiting, or trouble with balance should be checked out. Central nervous system tumors also frequently create vertigo and balance problems, visual changes, and other complications.

Remember that brain tumors are rare. Also, a brain tumor is not a death sentence. After treatment with surgery, chemotherapy, and/or radiation, many people with brain tumors go on to lead normal lives.

Meningitis

Meningitis is an inflammation of the membrane (meninges) that surrounds the brain and spinal cord. A bacteria or a virus causes this infection. One of the main symptoms of meningitis is a stiff neck. Other symptoms are a bad headache that doesn't go away, fever, lack of energy, or unconsciousness. Bacterial meningitis can be very serious, but treatment with specialized antibiotics usually cures the disease. Viral meningitis is usually not as serious as bacterial meningitis, and most patients recover without medication.

Viral Meningitis

One of the most common, and generally least dangerous, forms of meningitis is viral meningitis. Viral meningitis will normally clear up by itself without complications. Viral meningitis is sometimes called aseptic meningitis because analysis of the cerebrospinal fluid appears consistent with meningitis, but no bacterial cause is found. Nearly every aseptic meningitis is caused by a virus.

Many different viruses can cause meningitis, including herpes simplex types 1 and 2, mumps, influenza, Epstein-Barr, measles, rubella, and polio, among others. The most common causes of viral meningitis are enteroviruses. These viruses normally live in the intestines. Enteroviruses like Coxsackie and echovirus are often the cause of viral meningitis, especially in the summer and early fall. Since many people who have it do not get sick enough to seek medical attention, it is difficult to know how widespread

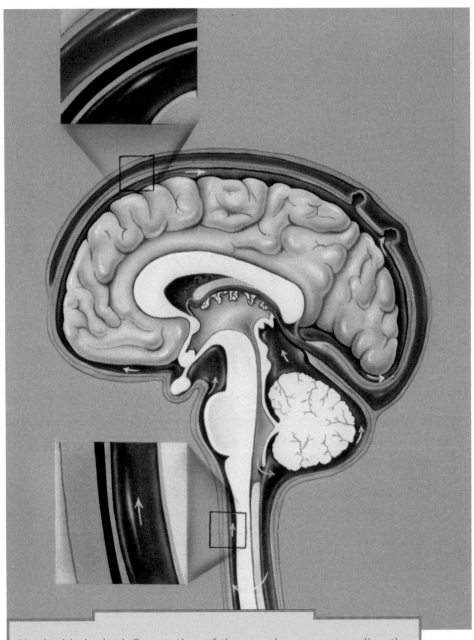

Meningitis is the inflammation of the membrane surrounding the brain and spinal cord, which are illustrated here.

viral meningitis might be. Statistics are available only for the cases severe enough to require hospitalization. With the exception of HSV meningitis, which is very serious in infant children, most viral meningitis goes away on its own.

In populations where vaccinations are common, some of these causes of meningitis are rare. In the United States, for instance, meningitis from the mumps would be extremely unusual. However, in unimmunized populations, a full 30 percent of the people who contract the mumps virus will develop viral meningitis. Strangely, males are two to five times more likely than females to develop viral meningitis in this way.

Other viruses that may cause meningitis include those spread by mosquitoes and ticks, like the St. Louis encephalitis virus, West Nile virus, the eastern equine encephalitis virus, and the Colorado tick fever virus.

Fungal Meningitis

Fungi can also cause meningitis. *Candida*, *Histoplasma*, coccidia, and *Cryptococcus* fungi have all been responsible for meningitis infections. Most cases of fungal meningitis occur in people who are already sick with a disease like AIDS, which has suppressed their immune systems. The fungi that cause meningitis are found in the environment and are spread by air currents. Healthy people with normal immune systems are extremely unlikely to ever develop fungal meningitis. Several of these fungi are found in soil, and others, like *Candida*, are found everywhere, including on human skin and inside the intestines.

Coccidioidal Meningitis

Meningitis caused by *Coccidioides immitis* is called coccidioidal meningitis. If left untreated, it is usually fatal. This fungus lives in the soil, and you can develop this infection by inhaling fungal particles into your lungs. It can be found in the southwestern United States, Mexico, and Central and South America. This fungus can also cause encephalitis, which is an infection of the brain itself.

Larval worms traveling throughout the human body can also cause meningitis. One worm that sometimes causes the disease

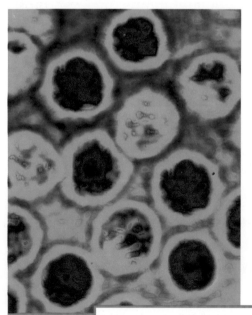

is *Strongyloides stercoralis*. It lives in tropical and subtropical areas. The adult worms live in the intestines, and their eggs are expelled from the body in the feces.

Once the eggs hatch, the new worms can enter a person through the skin. From there, they migrate to the lungs, travel to the throat, are swallowed, and develop into

Coccidioidal meningitis is caused by the fungus *Coccidioides immitis*, shown here.

adults inside the intestines. The worms can survive in the soil for several generations before they find a host.

Sometimes, these worms travel to other parts of the body, like the liver or the meninges. If they reach the meninges, the infected person can develop meningitis.

Exposure to soil that is contaminated with human feces is the main way to catch this parasite, which is more prevalent in tropical environments. The only way to keep people from being infected is to eliminate exposure to contaminated soil.

Rat Lungworm

Another worm that can cause problems is the rat lungworm, which is common only in Southeast Asia and the Pacific Islands. However, it has also been found in Puerto Rico, Africa, and Louisiana, and was probably brought to these places by infected rats arriving from foreign ports. The eggs leave the rat in feces and develop in an intermediate host like a snail, crab, or shrimp. Humans can get the worm from eating undercooked seafood. From the intestines, these worms can travel throughout the body, including to the meninges. Other worms that can infect such animals as dogs, cats, and raccoons are spread in the same way. You can acquire these worms by eating undercooked food and, rarely, by swimming in unclean water. The main way to avoid infection by parasites is to cook all food thoroughly, heating it to a high enough temperature to kill parasites.

Amoebas, which are single-celled organisms, can also cause parasitic meningitis. One of the species of amoebas that attacks humans is *Naegleria fowleri*. Amoebas invade the body through the nasal passages. This form of meningitis is called primary amebic meningoencephalitis. In its most serious form, primary amebic meningoencephalitis can kill a healthy person within seventy-two hours. To avoid this form of meningitis, people should not swim in fresh lakes, ponds, and rivers. Ensuring that swimming pools are properly chlorinated and that tap water has been treated adequately will also help to prevent this form of meningitis.

Other Forms of Meningitis

In rare cases, meningitis can be caused by chemical irritation (chemical meningitis) and tumors (carcinomatous meningitis). Although they are used infrequently, the chemicals responsible for chemical meningitis are often drugs like the ones administered to organ transplant recipients. In extremely rare circumstances, over-the-counter painkillers have been known to cause the inflammation, too.

Aneurysm

An aneurysm is a bulging, or weak, blood vessel. When an aneurysm leaks or bursts, it causes a hemorrhage, or severe bleeding. If a hemorrhage goes into or around the brain, the bleeding will cause great pain (a thunderclap headache). Also, as with meningitis, the bleeding will cause a stiff neck. If not treated by surgery, the aneurysm may cause unconsciousness or even death.

Severe Head Injuries

A severe head injury from an accident, fall, or physical abuse can also cause bleeding in the head. This can result in a bad

Chronic migraines and headaches can be caused by severe head injuries that result from such trauma as car accidents and falls.

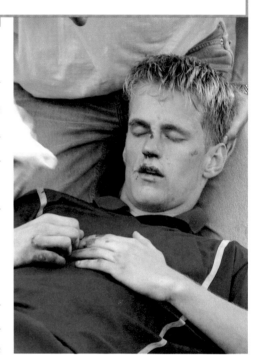

headache. Subdural bleeding is bleeding between the underside of the skull and the brain. A surgeon will have to drain the hemorrhage. This condition is a medical emergency.

Exertional Headaches

Exertion includes any kind of physical activity, even coughing. Exertion can cause headaches in some people.

Altitude Headaches

Until they become accustomed to the thinner air, people who go to places at high altitudes may experience headaches. Exertion, such as hiking or skiing, may make the headache worse. Altitude headaches cause a throbbing, pulsating pain. Pain relievers and increased oxygen sometimes help, but the best way to get rid of an altitude headache is to go back down the mountain.

Influenza and Other Viral or Bacterial Illnesses

Headaches often go hand in hand with various infections and fever. Bacteria and viruses produce headache-causing toxins (poisons). Fever can also cause headaches because of the increased blood flow to the brain and the dilation of the blood vessels.

Headaches from Substances

Some headaches are caused by ingesting or being exposed to certain substances. One common headache-causing food is ice cream, or rather the cold of the ice cream. However, an ice-cream headache usually lasts only a few seconds or minutes.

Drugs can cause much worse and longer-lasting headaches. Some of the drugs likely to cause headaches include alcohol, cocaine, and marijuana. Drinking too much alcohol causes many people to wake up the next morning with throbbing head pain. Drugs that raise the body's metabolism and blood pressure, such as cocaine, can even cause an aneurysm.

Carbon monoxide, often caused by faulty heaters or gas stoves, can also cause headaches. This headache can be a warning of danger to come. If the level of carbon monoxide in a person's blood rises to over 50 percent, the person may go into a coma and die. For protection, your family should have a carbon monoxide detector installed in your home. It is also

Ingesting certain substances, such as drugs, alcohol, or even too much coffee, can bring on migraines and headaches.

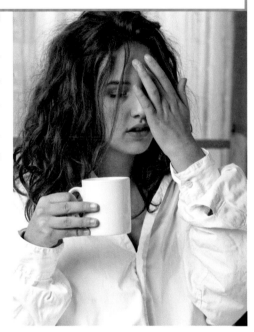

important to remember never to leave your garage door closed while a car is running inside since the carbon monoxide gets trapped inside and is often life-threatening.

Myths and Facts

 Sinus trouble causes migraine headaches.
Fact ➡ A sinus infection may cause a headache but probably not a migraine.

 Eye strain causes migraine headaches.
Fact ➡ Eye strain is unlikely to cause migraine headaches or other headaches.

 Allergies cause migraine headaches.
Fact ➡ A migraine headache is not an allergic reaction, and allergies are rarely a cause of migraine headaches.

 If you get a lot of migraine headaches, you probably have a brain tumor. Fact ➡ Brain tumors cause a very small percentage of headaches. Also, migraine headaches occur in cycles. A brain tumor usually causes a headache that gets progressively worse over time and is usually associated with other symptoms.

HOW DO YOU RECOGNIZE MIGRAINES?

Migraines and other headaches are scary. However, the more you know about your headaches, the better you will be able to deal with them. Steve Lindner, M.D., a pediatric neurologist in Dallas, Texas, says that most kids want to know three things about their headaches:

- What is the cause?
- What will make my headaches better?
- Are you sure I don't have a life-threatening illness?

Most people don't go to the doctor if they feel they don't have to. Even those with the most severe headaches tend to treat themselves with over-the-counter pain medications, or they just suffer. But when headaches start to interfere with your life, you need to get help.

Who Can Help?

As we have seen, medical conditions can contribute to headaches. When your head feels like it's ready to pop, you want instant relief, but you should first find out the cause of your headache. Medical practitioners are the best-equipped professionals to figure out your headache type and to offer appropriate remedies.

Your primary care physician may be a general practitioner, a family physician, or a pediatrician. It is helpful if this doctor is someone you have known over the years and feel comfortable

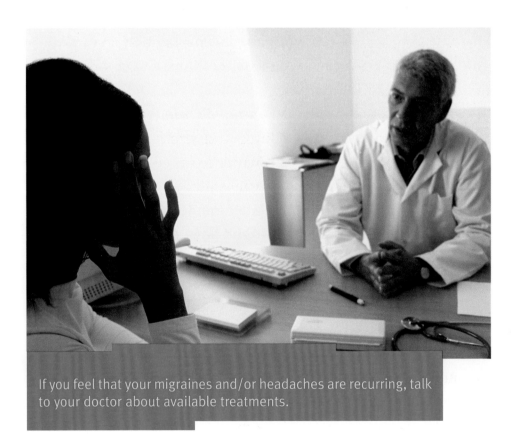

If you feel that your migraines and/or headaches are recurring, talk to your doctor about available treatments.

with. If your primary doctor can diagnose and treat your headaches, you may not have to see a specialist.

If, after a period of time, you do not get relief from your headaches, you may need to see a specialist. Your primary physician can refer you to a pediatric neurologist, who is a specialist in two disciplines: pediatrics (the care of young people) and neurology (the care of the brain, spinal cord, and nerves).

In addition to a primary doctor and/or a neurologist, you may also get help from a psychologist or psychiatrist. Both specialize in the ways emotions contribute to physical illness and the ways in which physical illnesses contribute to emotional distress. For example, a person who has frequent, severe migraines or chronic daily headaches may get depressed and feel that life with a constant headache is not worth living. Stress can cause headaches as well.

Psychologists and licensed clinical social workers can help manage your depressive feelings and stress. Psychiatrists are counselors, too. In addition, psychiatrists can prescribe medication to treat depression. A children's hospital or university hospital may also have a headache clinic. If you go to a headache clinic, your doctor will be a specialist who sees people with the most stubborn and hard-to-treat headaches.

Your Family's Headache History

One of the most important things a doctor does before making a diagnosis of migraine or other headache is to take a history. Your parents have known you your whole life, and they also know about their own parents. Because migraines tend to run in families, try to get both of your parents to go with you on your first visit to the doctor. However, if there are things that you would like to discuss in private, it's OK to ask to speak to the doctor alone. Before doing a physical examination, the doctor will ask questions such as:

- Who else in your family (on your mother's or father's side) has had migraines or other headaches? Do either of your parents have migraines? Do any of your siblings have headaches?
- Are any past or current events causing you extreme grief—death, divorce, family turmoil, or trouble in school or with friends?
- Have you had any significant illness? Are you taking any regular medications, drinking alcohol, or using any illegal substances?

Other questions a doctor might ask may be about your personal headache history, such as:

- How old do you think you were when you had your first headache?
- Have your headaches gotten better or worse since that first one?
- Have you noticed anything that seems to trigger a headache? A certain food? Bright light? Stress? Menstrual periods for females?
- At what time of day do you usually get a headache?

➤ What have you tried to cure your headaches? What works? What doesn't work?

➤ Are you worried about a more serious cause of your headaches, such as illness?

Getting a Physical Exam

The physical exam is important because it can rule out serious headache causes. A doctor will look in your eyes and test your balance and reflexes. These observations can tell a great deal about what is (or what is not) going on in your brain. To help a doctor diagnose the cause of your headaches, the doctor may use some of the following equipment:

➤ Computed tomography (CT) scans are also called computerized axial tomography (CAT) scans. These are fancy names for methods of taking a picture of your brain, also called neuroimaging. A neuroimaging system allows doctors to map cross sections of various parts of your body, including your brain. Scans are useful in detecting tumors, hemorrhages, and other serious causes of headaches.

➤ Magnetic resonance imaging (MRI) and magnetic resonance angiography (MRA) are both painless picture-taking procedures. The MRI uses powerful magnets to detect serious brain abnormalities, such as tumors and hemorrhages. The MRA is a similar procedure used to observe the large blood vessels of the head to see if there are abnormalities or obstructions.

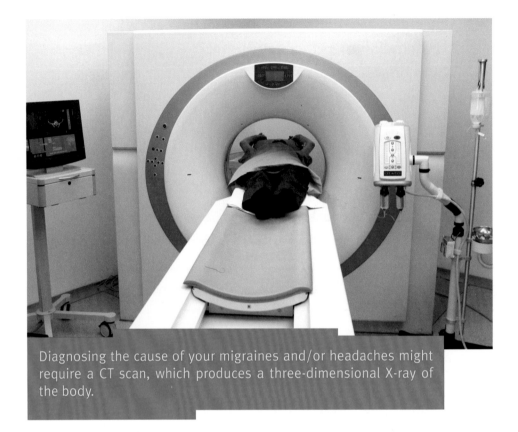

Diagnosing the cause of your migraines and/or headaches might require a CT scan, which produces a three-dimensional X-ray of the body.

→ Angiography is a more invasive procedure than MRI or MRA. A doctor inserts a small tube into a blood vessel. The tube is used to insert a dye into the blood vessel that shows if there has been a rupture.

→ An electrocardiogram (EEG) is usually not a part of a doctor's study of headaches. It is a painless procedure in which electrodes, attached to a patient's scalp, show unusual brain wave patterns. However, this is used more frequently to asses seizures.

→ A lumbar puncture or spinal tap, as it is sometimes called, is not necessary in routine headache testing. Its major use, though, is in diagnosing meningitis (infection of the linings of the brain) or encephalitis (infection of the brain itself).

How You Can Prepare for Your Doctor

As you may have guessed, reporting your condition honestly to your doctor is one of the most important parts of the migraine diagnosis. Now that you know some of the questions a doctor will ask, keep these questions in mind. Write down your "headache story." Make sure that the story you write down is honest. The personal story of your headaches, including when they started and what they are like, will be very helpful to the doctor who is trying to diagnose you. Be sure to bring your story to your first doctor visit.

The idea of a diary devoted exclusively to your headaches may not appeal to you. Some headaches are so bad that you wonder how you could ever forget them. However, as one headache merges into another, you may not remember as much as you expect. Do you remember exactly what stressed you on Monday, or at what time you ate chocolate on Tuesday? The answer to a memory problem is a precise headache diary.

Some doctors will give you a headache diary with a formatted table, but you can also make your own. Get a loose-leaf notebook and fill it with the following categories:

- Day and date
- When headache began and ended
- Warning signs
- Other symptoms

Help your doctor out by keeping track of your headache history. Document when you get them, how severe they are, and how long they last.

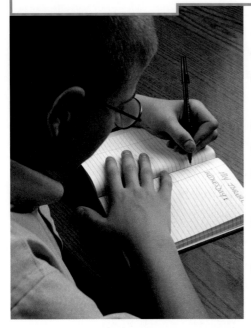

➤ Medications taken

➤ Things that helped you feel better

➤ Location of headache

➤ Type of pain

➤ Intensity of pain on a scale of 1 to 10

➤ What you ate or drank pre-headache

➤ Unusual events or stressors

Keep your headache diary as faithfully as you can and for as long as you can. Be sure to take your headache diary to your doctor. Together, the two of you can try to find headache patterns and contributing factors. Above all, be honest with yourself and your doctor.

Ten Great Questions to Ask Your Doctor

1 How will migraines impact me at home, at school, and with my friends?

2 What are the best treatment options for me?

3 What can I do to avoid getting a migraine?

4 When I do get a migraine, is there anything else I can do to relieve the pain besides taking my medicine?

5 Will I always get migraines or will I outgrow them?

6 Are there certain foods that trigger migraines?

7 What do I do if my headache continues after taking my medicines?

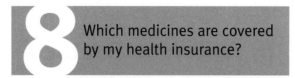

8 Which medicines are covered by my health insurance?

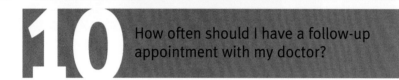

9 What are the signs that my headaches are not under control with the medicines I am taking?

10 How often should I have a follow-up appointment with my doctor?

HOW DO I PREVENT MIGRAINES?

When it comes to headache prevention, there is good news and bad news. The bad news is that preventing headaches is not always possible. The good news is that prevention is worth a try since many people find out that it works. Work on the lifestyle changes listed here. They certainly won't hurt and they may help. (Medications for headache prevention are listed last because doctors prescribe them only for frequent and stubborn headaches.)

Avoiding Headache Triggers

Various influences combine to produce a headache. Headache "triggers" are internal or external forces that contribute to migraines in susceptible people. One person's triggers may not even bother another person. The goal is to determine your personal triggers.

See if exercising three or four times a week for at least twenty minutes a day boosts your headache-prevention threshold. Running, swimming, and playing basketball are all excellent ways to exercise, and doing activities that you enjoy will make you more likely to continue.

Avoiding stress is easier said than done. In fact, it's nearly impossible to avoid stress completely. The important thing is how you react to stress. You may have already found your own ways to relax. Listening to music is one way; talking with friends is another. Experts also suggest the following techniques. Try some of them and see if they work for you.

Imagery and/or visualization: Once a headache has taken hold, it may be too late to use imagery or visualization. Regularly practice seeing yourself in a relaxing setting, free of stress. Close your eyes and imagine yourself on a quiet beach. You hear no sounds, except for the crash of waves against the shore. Inhale. Smell the salty ocean air. Imagine the heat of the sun on your shoulders and the burning sand under your feet. To make visualization even easier, get a tape or CD with relaxing music and directions to guide you.

Conscious breathing: Breathing is something we do twenty-four hours a day, but we don't usually give it much thought. Try paying attention to your breath. (Concentrating on your breath is one of many types of meditation.) Wearing comfortable clothes, sit in a chair in a quiet place. Inhale and count slowly to three. Exhale. Pay attention only to your breathing. Keep up this conscious inhaling and exhaling for several minutes.

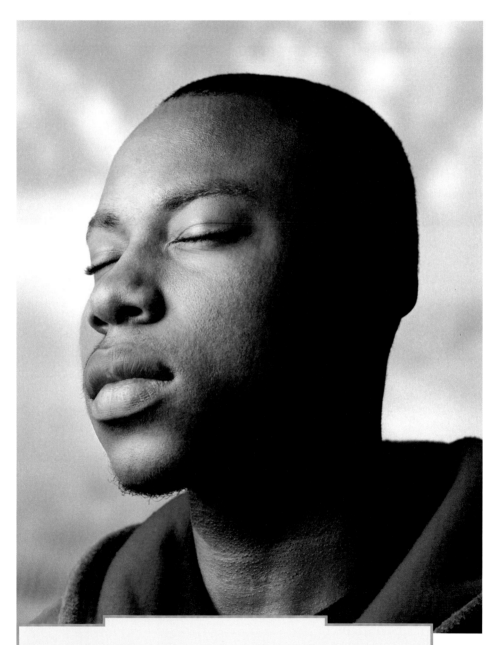

Relaxation and meditation are great, natural ways to relieve, or even prevent, headaches.

Progressive muscle relaxation: Lie on the floor or on a bed. The idea is to squeeze every voluntary muscle in your body, hold the squeeze for a few seconds, and then relax. Start with your head, the source of your misery. Squeeze your eyebrows together into a frown. Hold that pose as long as you can, then relax. Then, squeeze your eyes tightly shut. Relax. Next, scrunch up your nose like a rabbit. Hold it. Relax. Get the idea? Move down your body, tensing and relaxing every muscle you can think of.

Laugh: Studies show that laughter helps to relieve stress. In the middle of a migraine, you may not feel much like laughing.

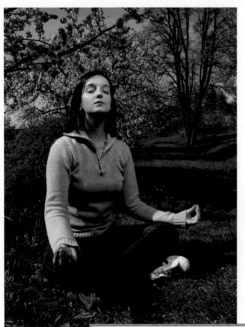

But in your headache-free periods, get in the humor habit. Watch funny movies. Make someone else laugh and laugh with them. Laughing relaxes your face muscles and is good exercise.

Yoga: Yoga is a very popular form of relaxation that helps to relieve anxiety and stress. It is an ancient system of exercises, postures, stretches,

Yoga has shown to be an excellent, nonmedicinal way to relieve headache stress.

breathing, and meditation. You can learn yoga in a class or individually with an instructor.

Tai chi chuan (tai chi): Tai chi, a Chinese martial art, is sometimes used to relieve stress and to encourage healing. It involves slow, graceful body movements. *Chi* is the Chinese term for the body's vital energy force. You can do tai chi by yourself or in a group.

Grades, activities, and other aspects of school life can cause distress for teens. The following are some of the issues that all teens deal with during their school years:

Grades

Getting good grades was one of the top five school stressors listed by teens in several surveys. The push for good grades is often driven by things other than the love of learning. In order to participate in most sports programs and be recruited to play college sports, students must maintain high grade-point averages.

Teens also believe that being admitted to top schools depends on getting high grades. They are correct. Good high school grades, difficulty of a student's high school course selection, and scores on SAT or ACT exams are among the most important factors for college admission.

Being accepted to a prestigious university is important to teens who are concerned about future earning power. They believe a degree from a famous school will help them get a higher-paying job when they graduate.

Activity Overload

Activity overload is another source of stress for teens. It takes more than grades for a teen to get into a good college or university. But how much more? College admission committees look at students' extracurricular activities to get a feel for what their interests are. Teens may be carrying the push to appear well-rounded too far. Many are packing so much into their lives that they are truly stressed out. Learning to say no diplomatically is difficult, but it is perhaps one of the greatest skills one can learn.

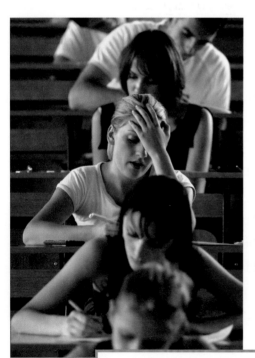

Deciding on Colleges

Making decisions about which college to attend, or whether to go to college at all, is stressful for many teens. Should you try for a certain college because "that's where Mom/Dad went"? Should you follow your friends to the local community college? Should you

One way to avoid migraines and headaches is to try to stem the stress in your life. Balance your schoolwork with less taxing activities such as hobbies and socializing.

apply to ten colleges or two? All of these questions weigh heavily on teens, even those still in middle school. While bucking parental expectations and peer pressure in making decisions about college may create stress, doing what you really want to do may be worth it.

Many teens feel a great amount of stress in dealing with their peers. Dating, fitting in, and handling conflicts with peers are among the most stressful situations that can confront teenagers today.

Herbs, Vitamins, and Minerals

If you want to try natural remedies for the prevention of migraines, be sure to check with your doctor first to make sure they are safe. Excessive doses of some herbal substances can do more harm than good. For example, high doses of vitamin A can actually cause headaches.

Another common herb used to treat migraines is feverfew. However, people who are allergic to the sunflower family (ragweed, chrysanthemum, marigolds, daisies) should avoid this herb.

Another herbal supplement is called 5-HPT. This is derived from the seeds of an African plant, *Griffonia simplicifolia*. This supplement has many possible side effects, and people with liver trouble should not use it.

Natural remedies may be best for some people, but even natural remedies have a potential for harm. Herbal remedies can cause side effects and may have a negative interaction with other drugs.

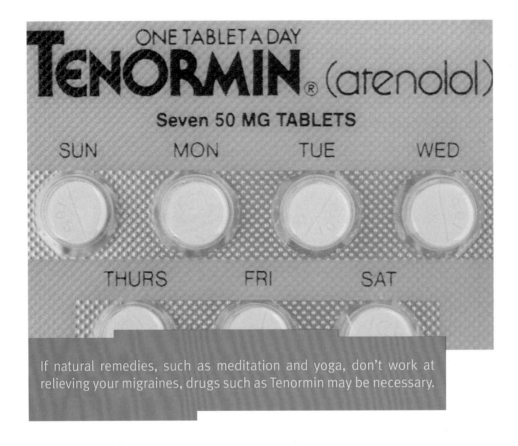

If natural remedies, such as meditation and yoga, don't work at relieving your migraines, drugs such as Tenormin may be necessary.

Migraine Prevention Medications

Ask yourself these questions:

- Do I have more than two migraine headaches a month?
- Do I have migraines that severely disrupt my life?
- Are the medications I am taking to relieve my headaches ineffective?

If you answered yes to any of the questions above, your doctor may be willing to prescribe preventive medications. It is up to you whether you want to take a pill every day. Sometimes, after taking preventive medication for about six months or so, your doctor will help you to taper off the medication. Many people are able to stay off it for good.

The following medications are commonly used for young people. They are safe when prescribed by a medical doctor. They are listed with their scientific names first. The trade names are in parentheses.

Teens sometimes have good luck with small doses of tricyclic antidepressants, such as amitriptyline (Elavil). Another helpful class of preventive drugs are beta blockers. Doctors originally used these medications to control high blood pressure. They help to prevent migraine headaches by stabilizing the blood vessels and regulating blood flow to the brain. Examples of these medications are propranolol (Inderal), nadolol (Corgard), and atenolol (Tenormin).

There is help available for migraine sufferers, and new drugs are appearing every year. Medication, in combination with wellness strategies, can greatly reduce the suffering caused by migraine headaches.

HOW SHOULD I TREAT MIGRAINES?

Just as headaches are divided into categories, so is treatment. We can divide headache treatment into medicinal—or treatments using medication—and nonmedicinal. There are benefits and drawbacks to both medicinal and non-medicinal treatments depending on the severity of your condition. Only a doctor can determine which is the best course of action for you, but what follows is a rundown of each.

Medicinal Migraine Treatment

In considering treatment for your headaches, a doctor may prescribe medicines that will relieve accompanying symptoms as well as the pain in your head. Be sure to start out taking the smallest amount of medication that works.

Nonprescription Medications

A doctor will probably suggest that you first try nonprescription (over-the-counter) medications. Take them at the first sign of a headache. These include acetaminophen (Tylenol) or ibuprofen (Advil, Nuprin, or Motrin). People under the age of fifteen should not use aspirin because of the danger of Reye's syndrome, an illness that causes severe vomiting and possibly coma. Other types of headache relievers are the nonsteroidal anti-inflammatory drugs (NSAIDs). These include naproxen sodium, sold over the counter as Aleve.

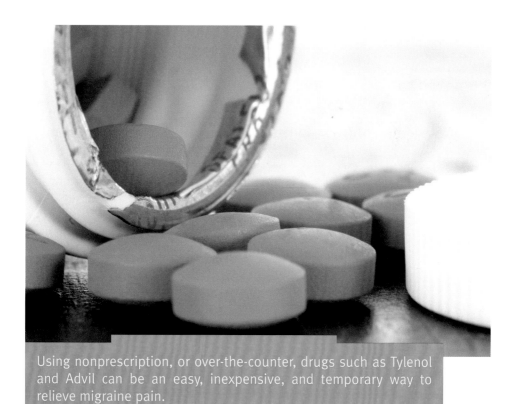

Using nonprescription, or over-the-counter, drugs such as Tylenol and Advil can be an easy, inexpensive, and temporary way to relieve migraine pain.

Prescription Medications

It is likely that you will need to take several different medicines depending on the type and severity of your migraines. If you need something to relieve the nausea and vomiting caused by your migraines, the doctor may prescribe antiemetics. These are able to be taken by mouth (for nausea), by suppository (in case of vomiting), or by intravenous injection (IV). For a full-blown headache, doctors sometimes prescribe a combination drug. You and your doctor can work together to find the best medicines for treating your headaches.

Nonmedicinal Treatments

It is possible to get some relief from migraines with nonmedicinal treatments. These treatments are not likely to cure a migraine on their own, but they may make someone suffering from a migraine more comfortable.

➤ **Sleep:** Sleep is one of the most effective treatments for migraine headaches. For some people, a nap or a full night's sleep is all that is needed to beat the pain.
➤ **Ice:** An ice pack on your aching head will probably not cure your headache, but it may make it feel better for a while.
➤ **Exercise:** Exercise may seem like the opposite of relaxation, but many people find that exercise helps to calm them down. Exercise can make some headaches worse, but for other headaches, exercise is a pain reliever.

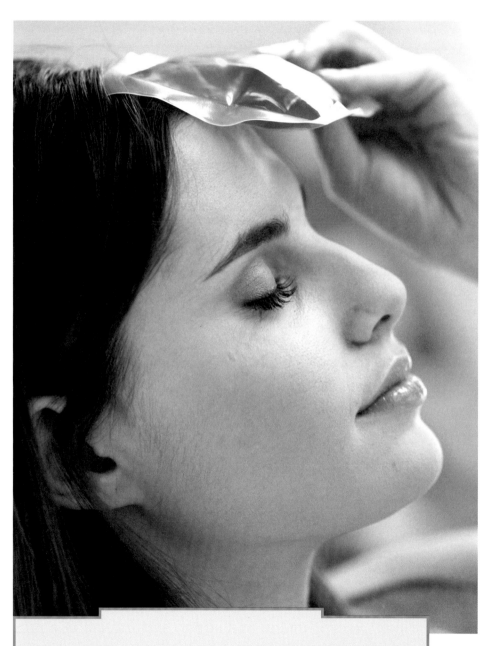

Simple cures, such as placing an ice pack on your forehead, can be helpful in relieving pain.

➤ **Massage:** A massage always feels good, especially to those with tension or chronic daily headaches. You don't need a professional massage. Find someone who is willing to rub your neck and head muscles. Touch is a powerful pain reliever.

Controlling Stress

The teen years are a time of major life crises. You are experiencing physical changes that are stressful, developing your own beliefs and values, and developing relationships that may be long lasting. You have endless demands on your time and are bombarded by new challenges every day. No wonder you are stressed! As you have seen, there are many contributing factors to stress and several negative ways to deal with stress that often only compound our stress. Perhaps some of the positive coping mechanisms presented here will prove to be helpful. Underlying all of these is one recurring theme—you are not alone. Regardless of what your stressors are and how hopeless things may seem, talking with someone will help. Give it a try.

Dealing with stress in a positive manner can be hard work. Here are suggestions that will help you develop positive coping mechanisms.

Learn to Like Yourself

Having a positive self-image and strong self-esteem is a prerequisite for developing positive coping skills. How do you improve your self-image and boost your self-esteem? The first

> Overall, the best way to feel good physically and mentally is to have a positive outlook on life.

step is to list things you like about yourself. As you do that, you will undoubtedly think of things you don't like about yourself. The second step is to change the things you don't like. Start with changes that are easy to make, like getting a new hairstyle or a few new clothes. Take a positive approach to things that are harder to change—your

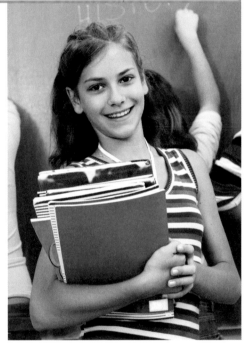

weight, for instance. Think of these changes as challenges rather than obstacles.

As you improve your self-image, you will start to improve your self-esteem. Here are other ways to strengthen your self-esteem:

- Use positive self-speak. You constantly have mental conversations with yourself. If you bad-mouth yourself, you soon start to believe you are a bad person. Put a positive spin on your self-conversations.

➤ Be tolerant of your own mistakes. Nobody is perfect. It is easy to be excessively critical of yourself. If you make a mistake, admit that you did, learn from the experience, and then let it go.

➤ Acknowledge your accomplishments. Make a habit of recognizing even the smallest of your accomplishments every day. Make a list of them—even if they don't seem very important. By recognizing and being proud of your accomplishments, you begin to understand your self-worth.

➤ Be assertive. Being able to let others know what you think and feel is important. After all, what you have to say is just as important as what others have to say. So, say what you think, but also listen to others and respect their opinions.

➤ Spend time with people who value you. The people you choose to be around are often mirrors of how you feel about yourself. If the people you hang around with are constantly putting you down, you're running with the wrong crowd!

Take Control

With your self-image buffed and your self-esteem maximized, you are ready to deal with stress and make it work for you. Here are a few steps to help you take control:

Define the Problem

Making plans to deal with stress is difficult if you don't know what is causing it. Spend several days jotting down things that cause you stress. Then, make a definitive list of your major stressors. Just recognizing a stressor may actually make it less stressful.

Learn to Manage Time

One of the main stressors identified by teens is the lack of time to do everything that is expected of them. True, teens are busy, but much of the problem lies in poor time management. Make daily and weekly schedules to manage your time more efficiently. Start by listing daily and weekly activities you absolutely must do, like classes, band practice, and student council meetings, for example. After you get all of the "must dos" into your schedule, fill in some of the uncommitted time slots with things you should do, like getting started on the research for a term paper. You are in charge of the schedule, so build time into it for everything, including "alone" time, family time, etc. Keep this schedule with you so you can update it as needed. No schedule is perfect, but if you stick with it most of the time, you will find even an incredibly busy schedule to be must less stressful than it was before.

Learn to Say No

Most people agree to do a lot of things they really don't want to do simply because they think they should. Some of these are unavoidable, especially those that your parents and teachers ask you to do, but others are not. Rather than agreeing immediately to being on another committee or participating in another after school activity, think about your motivation for doing so. If you really have no interest in the activity or time for it, say no. Guard your time—no one else will.

Practice and Prepare

One of the most stressful things you can do is to approach an event without being prepared. If you always wait until the last minute to prepare a speech or study for a test, you will be under a lot more stress than if you prepare ahead of time. By being prepared, you can harness your stress and make it work for you.

Finish What You Start

You can minimize stress by making a concerted effort to finish each project or chore as it comes along, rather than putting it off. Break big chores into a group of smaller tasks that can be completed in a reasonable time. Soon the entire project will be done, and you will get a great deal of satisfaction from checking it off of your list.

Be Good to Your Body

Coping with outside stressors if you are physically stressed is very difficult. The "big three" of staying physically healthy are: eat right, get enough sleep, and get plenty of exercise.

Eat Right

Stress reactions require your body to expend tremendous amounts of energy. Where do you get this energy? From food, of course. Fast food, snacks, and sodas won't hack it. They are high in calories, fats, and caffeine, and low in basic nutrients, vitamins, and minerals. Take the time to eat well-rounded meals and save the junk food for occasional treats. Your body also needs a lot of water to keep its systems working. Most teens do not drink enough fluids and border on being dehydrated much of the time. Extreme tiredness, crankiness, slight nausea, and faintness are some signs of dehydration. They can be corrected quickly by simply drinking water.

Get Enough Sleep

How much is enough? Most people need between seven and eight hours of sleep each night. Few get that much sleep. Teens tend to fall asleep later at night and, if their schedules allow, sleep later in the morning than do adults or young children. If, however, they can't sleep late, they may become sleep deprived. Sleep deprivation leads to impairment in judgment and the ability to think, and may also lead to impairment in motor skills and reaction times. This can have serious consequences, especially if sleep-deprived teens are driving.

Get Plenty of Exercise

Exercise can decrease stress by causing increased production of endorphins, which are natural opioids found in the brain. This gives a natural "high" to counterbalance the lows of stress. Exercise is also an outlet for all the pent-up energy that stress produces. By expending the energy productively, you are less likely to react impulsively and violently in stressful situations.

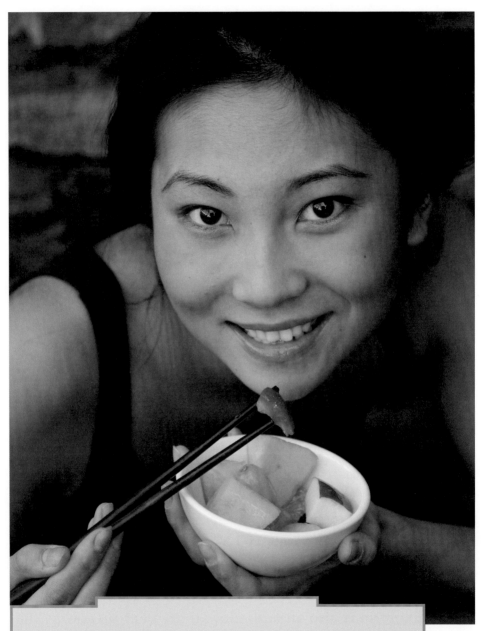

Getting exercise and eating right may be the most effective way to live a migraine-free life.

Researchers are making new headache treatments available all the time. Just remember that neither medical science nor alternative practitioners have discovered a headache cure. Yet, with a combination of prevention and treatment methods tailored specifically for you, you can get headache relief.

Glossary

aneurysm A widening of the walls of a blood vessel that may rupture.

antibiotic Medication that inhibits the growth of bacteria.

aura Sensory experiences, such as sparkling lights, that appear for some people thirty to sixty minutes before a migraine headache begins.

hemiparesis A weakness on one side of the body.

hemiplegia Paralysis on one side of the body.

meningitis Inflammation of the outer layer of the brain.

MRI (magnetic resonance imaging) A procedure that uses a magnetic field and radio waves to detect disease.

prodrome An early warning period before the onset of a migraine.

suppository Medicine in a form that can be inserted into the rectum for absorption.

trigger Anything that sets off a headache, including food, beverages, environmental conditions, psychological stressors, hormonal changes, or changes in one's normal routine.

For More Information

American Headache Society Committee for Headache
    Education (ACHE)
19 Mantua Road
Mount Royal, NJ 08061
(800) 255-ACHE (2243)
E-mail: achehq@talley.com
Web site: http://www.achenet.org
  ACHE is a nonprofit organization that works with
  patients and doctors to help people participate in their
  own care. The organization publishes a quarterly
  newsletter, *Headache*; helps to organize support groups;
  and offers support services online.

Insight Meditation Society
1230 Pleasant Street
Barre, MA 01005
Web site: http://www.dharma.org/ims
  One of the longest established meditation societies in the
  West, known for its down-to-earth style and silent medi-
  tation retreats.

Iyengar Yoga National Association of the United States
3010 Hennepin Ave. S, #272
Minneapolis, MN 55408

(800) 889-YOGA (9642)

Web site: http://www.iynaus.org

This association is dedicated to spreading the ideas and techniques of yogi guru B. K. S. Iyengar, who developed a unique yoga style that is particularly suitable for those practicing yoga despite physical challenges or limitations.

Jivamukti Yoga Center

404 Lafayette Street, 3rd Floor

New York, NY 10003

(800) 295-6814

Web site: http://www.jivamuktiyoga.com

This is the largest yoga center in the United States and is particularly focused on teaching yoga philosophy and history as well as physical asanas. Instructional CDs and DVDs are offered in addition to classes and teacher training courses.

Kripalu Yoga Center for Yoga and Health

P.O. Box 793 West Street, Route 183

Lenox, MA 01240

(866) 200-5204

Web site: http://www.kripalu.org

This is one of the largest yoga centers on the East Coast of the United States, and it investigates many different philosophies, techniques, and approaches in order to find better ways to help its students.

National Headache Foundation (NHF)

428 West Saint James Place, 2nd Floor

Chicago, IL 60614-2750

(800) 843-2256

Web site: http://www.headaches.org

The oldest and largest organization for those with headaches, the NHF is a volunteer, nonprofit group that provides free information about headaches; sends out lists of doctors who are members of the foundation; publishes a quarterly newsletter, *NHF Head Lines*; and can provide localized lists of support groups. If there are no support groups available in a person's area, the NHF can help interested persons start one.

National Institute of Neurological Disorders and Stroke (NINDS)

31 Center Drive MSC 2540

Building 31, Room 8A-06

Bethesda, MD 20892-2540

(800) 352-9424

E-mail: nindswebadmin@nih.gov

Web site: http://www.ninds.nih.gov

An agency of the United States federal government, this organization is the leading supporter of biomedical research on the brain and nervous system.

San Francisco Zen Center

300 Page Street

San Francisco, CA 94102

Web site: http://www.sfzc.org

A cornerstone of Zen Buddhism in America, this center was founded by the great Zen master Shunryu Suzuki Roshi in 1962. The site contains many links to Soto Zen communities.

Shambhala International
1084 Tower Road
Halifax, NS B3H 2Y5
Canada
Web site: http://www.shambhala.org
   An international network of meditation centers, founded by
   the great Tibetan teacher Chogyam Trungpa Rinpoche. The
   Shambhala Center nearest you will be a great resource as
   you begin on your path.

Springwater Center
7179 Mill Street
Springwater, NY 14560
Web site: http://www.springwatercenter.org
   This center was founded by Toni Packer, a former Zen
   Buddhist who decided to move away from the rituals of Zen
   practice. Here you will find a fresh and intelligent approach
   to the practice of meditation.

Web Sites

Due to the changing nature of Internet links, Rosen Publishing
has developed an online list of Web sites related to the subject
of this book. This site is updated regularly. Please use this link
to access the list:

http://www.rosenlinks.com/faq/mige

Diamond, Seymour, and Amy Diamond. *Headache and Your Child: The Complete Guide to Understanding and Treating Migraine and Other Headaches in Children and Adolescents.* New York, NY: Simon and Schuster, 2001.

Diamond, Seymour, and Mary A. Franklin. *Conquering Your Migraine: The Essential Guide to Understanding and Treating Migraines for All Sufferers and Their Families.* New York, NY: Simon and Schuster, 2001.

Johnson, Michael L. *What Do You Do When the Medications Don't Work? A Non-Drug Treatment of Dizziness, Migraine Headaches, Fibromyalgia, and Other Chronic Conditions.* Appleton, WI: Jokamar-Jenake Publishing, 2003.

Marks, David R., and Laura Marks. *The Headache Prevention Cookbook: Eating Right to Prevent Migraines and Other Headaches.* Boston, MA: Houghton Mifflin, 2000.

Mauskop, Alexander, and Barry Fox. *What Your Doctor May Not Tell You About Migraines: The Breakthrough Program That Can Help End Your Pain.* New York, NY: Warner Books, 2000.

Roberts, Teri. *Living Well with Migraine Disease and Headaches: What Your Doctor Doesn't Tell You . . . That You Need to Know.* New York, NY: Collins, 2005.

Stafford, Diane, and Jennifer Shoquist. *Migraines for Dummies.* Hoboken, NJ: Wiley, 2003.

Young, William B., Stephen D. Silberstein, and Austin J. Sumner. *Migraine and Other Headaches.* New York, NY: Demos Medical Publishing, 2006.

Index

About the Author

Allan Cobb is a writer and editor living in central Texas. He has written numerous young adult books related to medicine, including *The Bionic Human, First Responders, Heroin and Your Veins*, and *Scientifically Engineered Food: The Debate Over What's on Your Plate.*

Photo Credits

Cover, pp. 38, 40, 45, 49, 54 Shutterstock.com; p. 5 © www.istockphoto.com/Daniel Rodriguez; p. 11 © Dr. G. Ravily/ Photo Researchers, Inc.; p. 13 © www.istockphoto.com/Sal Sen; p. 16 © Bryson Biomedical Illustrations/Custom Medical Stock Photo; p. 18 © J. Cavallini/Custom Medical Stock Photo; p. 21 © www.istockphoto.com/Marjan Laznik; p. 23 © www.istockphoto. com/Paul Piebinga; p. 26 © BSIP/Phototake; p. 30 © www.istock-photo.com / Millanovic; p. 32 © Altrendo Images/Getty Images; p. 37 © James Ross/Getty Images; p. 42 © Custom Medical Stock Photo; p. 47 © GARO/Photo Researchers, Inc.

Designer: Evelyn Horovicz; Editor: Nicholas Croce